SHIATSU FOR DOGS

CONTENTS

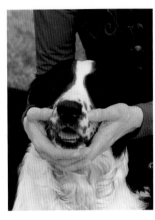

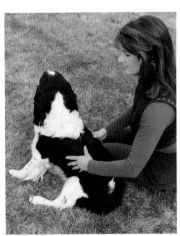

INTRODUCTION

THE BENEFITS OF TREATMENT

Giving shiatsu treatments to your dog will help you to get to know and communicate with him and to recognise what is and what is not the 'norm', thus signals of pain will be more apparent to you. Never force the treatments and techniques on your dog, his needs must always come first.

It becomes easy to detect changes in the muscles and joints because you are literally more in touch with the dog's body. By routinely moving each limb through range-of-motion exercises, less than fluid movement will seem quite obvious to both partners.

Muscular stress due to activity should diminish and disappear in a matter of days and a few shiatsu sessions. If not, and it becomes necessary to consult a vet, your experience with your dog's body will enable you to give a much more clear and detailed description of the ailment. Your vet will find it easier to perform an examination because the dog is accustomed to being handled.

Injuries will heal faster because circulation is improved.

Dogs become more aware of their bodies as they experience the pressure, stretching, and passive non-habitual movements during treatment time. The treatments will relax and calm dogs.

All dogs, whatever their situation or training will benefit both physically and mentally from shiatsu treatments.

LENGTH OF EACH TREATMENT

The duration of the treatment may be from five minutes up to one hour. Longer than this is too long. Half an hour is recom-

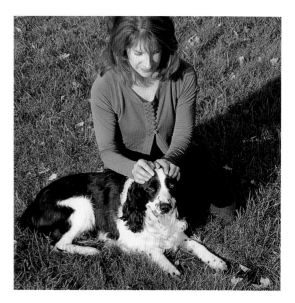

mended for a general full body session. I prefer to work for a shorter length of time. Five minutes may be enough and working only the back may be the entire treatment.

At any time during a session your dog may decide he has had enough, or just need a break. If he doesn't return in a short time, wait until next time.

AFTER THE TREATMENT

Keep your dog from leaping up and becoming active for about five minutes. This will help him experience a deeper relaxation than usual and let the benefits of your work take hold. Don't feed him immediately after a treatment.

Watch your dog carefully when he moves

WHAT NOT TO TREAT

Areas of broken skin – open wounds – areas that have been stitched or areas near these locations – inflamed joints where heat can be felt – broken bones.

Always consult your vet if your dog is injured or displaying extreme personality changes.

about. You may notice more graceful movements, more curiosity about his surroundings, and affectionate behaviour.

YOUR PREPARATION

Wear loose comfortable clothing and no watches or jewellery that may get caught in the dog's hair. Warm your hands. Prepare a quiet area, free from distractions. If working indoors, place a towel or blanket on the floor for you and your dog. Lighting should be soft. Try to work outside if possible.

Place your hands on your dog and take a few deep breaths to calm and centre yourself. Encourage your dog to sit or lie quietly, with your hands and your voice. Let him hear your deep rhythmic breathing as you work.

Begin the same way each time so your dog understands that this is a special time.

Finish by holding his body with both hands for a quiet moment together. Quietly move away.

THE BACK

Some dogs may accept the pressure along the back muscles while lying down, some may like to sit, some may prefer to stand.

It is quite usual for a dog to begin by receiving a shiatsu treatment while sitting. He might not want to lie down immediately but probably will do so eventually when he relaxes.

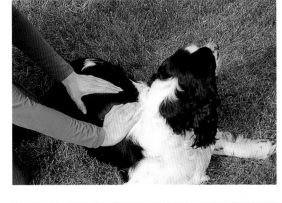

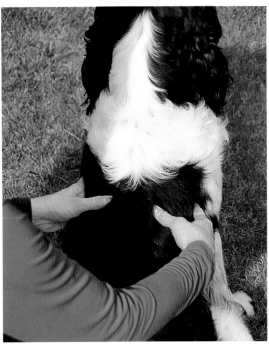

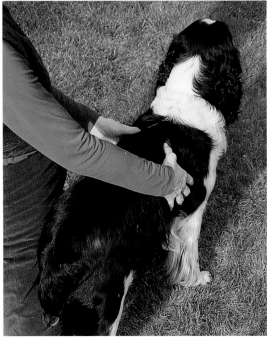

Press directly inward with your thumbs by moving your body towards the dog. Hold steadily for 3-5 seconds, and slowly release. Move smoothly to the next area, an inch or two downward from your previous contact point.

Work from the shoulders towards the tail; repeat two or three times in the same direction, supporting with your fingers on the sides of his body as you work. No pressure is applied directly to the spine, only to the muscles alongside the spine.

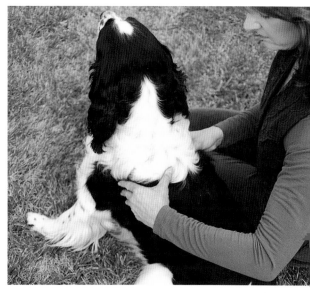

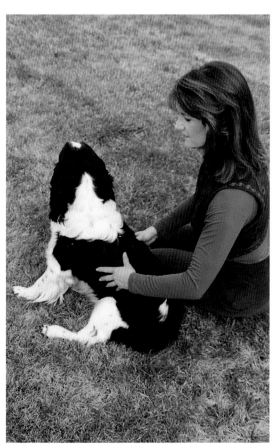

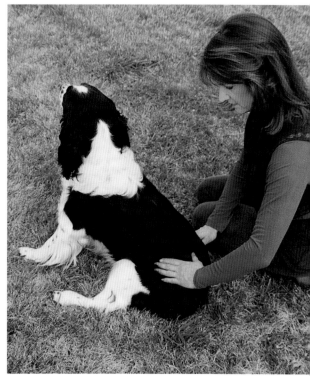

CORRECT BREATHING

During treatment, breathe low into your abdomen, letting it expand as you breathe in, relaxing as you breathe out. The exhalation is a bit slower than the inhalation. Keep your shoulders relaxed, and your facial features soft. Let your dog occasionally hear you breathe deeply. He may imitate you, or even remind you to breathe by taking a deep breath and sighing himself.

BACK STRETCHES

Give a gentle stretch by separating your hands: hold one behind the shoulders, the other in front of the hips, and lean your body forward. The pressure, which goes towards the head and the tail, creates a gentle stretch. Hold for 5-10 seconds, release slowly.

For a slightly stronger stretch, cross your arms, bring your body gradually toward his back. Hold for 5-10 seconds, release slowly.

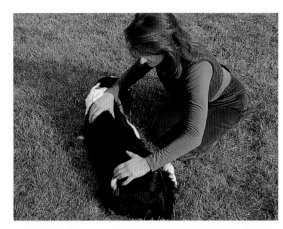

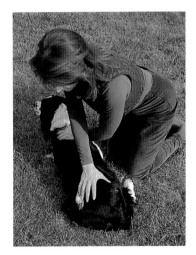
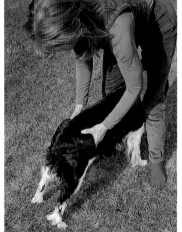
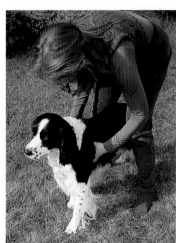

With your knees behind his shoulders and your hands holding him in the hip area, gently lean into your hands to create a stretch that will affect the back and sides. Hold for 5-10 seconds, release slowly. *OR*

reverse your position, secure his back end with your legs but do not press or squeeze. Apply your hands behind his shoulders and lean forward, creating a similar stretch. Hold for 5-10 seconds, release slowly.

STRETCHING TECHNIQUES

When practising a stretch, remember that the area to be stretched should have been warmed up first, either by pressure points, or rotations, and preferably both.

Bring the body part into its stretch position only to the point of slight resistance, and hold it there for a few seconds. Release it back to a relaxed position. Repeat the stretch, this time after holding in the stretched position for a few seconds, stretch a tiny bit further. Don't force this movement, just lean in slightly, moving the leg, for example perhaps a quarter of an inch. Hold for 5-10 seconds and very slowly bring it into a relaxed position.

Our goal is not to increase the range of motion each time but to keep a normal range of motion, free and unrestricted.

You must remember to exhale as you make each stretch in order to keep yourself relaxed.

SHOULDER ROTATION

Sit comfortably and embrace the top of the leg with relaxed hands. Move your body to accomplish a smooth circular rotation.

Move from a neutral position (1) to the rear (2) upwards (3) forwards and downwards (4). This creates a range of shoulder rotation motion, without force or strain. Repeat two or three times in each direction. Each complete movement may take 5-10 seconds.

ROTATION TECHNIQUES

When rotating a joint, always support the area with both hands and work with a circular movement, either clockwise or counter clockwise. Stay relaxed and lean your body into the rotation as if you were part of the shoulder, hip or any area that moves. Move your body first, using no force or muscular power.

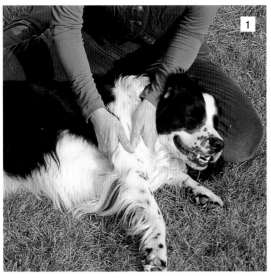
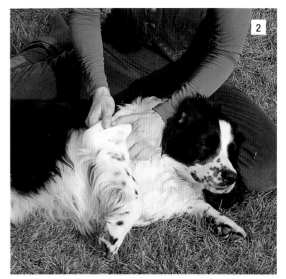
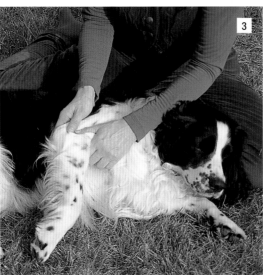
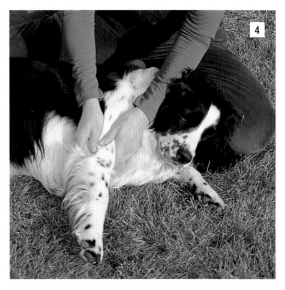

FRONT LEG STRETCH

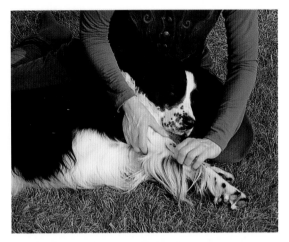

FORWARD

Support the leg with one hand on or just below the shoulder. Using the fingertips of the other hand, apply gentle pressure down the leg, holding each location for a few seconds as you work your way towards the foot. During this process, you may begin to lean your body slightly to the side, to create the beginning of a stretch.

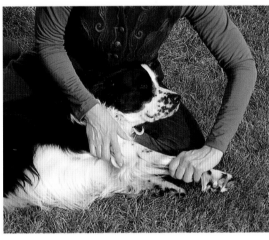

Holding just above the foot and behind the shoulder, slowly lean your body to the side, creating a long gentle stretch. Breathe out as you go into the stretch. Don't squeeze the leg, just hold it firmly enough to give support. Hold for 5-10 seconds, then bring the leg back into a neutral position.

The stretch illustrated below may be done sitting in front of the dog. Support the leg and stretch by slowly leaning backwards, then release gradually.

FACIAL EXPRESSIONS

During all movement techniques, watch your dog's facial expression for reactions to what you are doing. If he seems to be at all insecure, go back to a technique that was more comfortable. Do not attempt to increase range of motion, rather support existing capabilities.

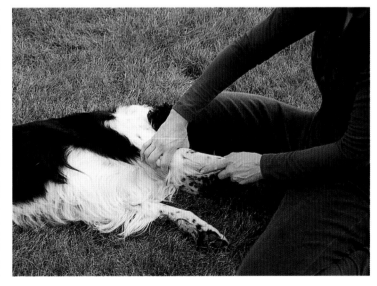

REARWARD

Support the upper leg with one hand and press along the front of the leg with the thumb of the other hand. Take the leg gradually rearwards as you press along the leg at regular intervals from shoulder to foot. Hold each location for a few seconds. If any points seem painful, release pressure and return the leg to a neutral position.

When you have reached the foot, hold, then lean your body gently forwards to take the leg into a stretch. Hold for 5-10 seconds and return the leg to a neutral position.

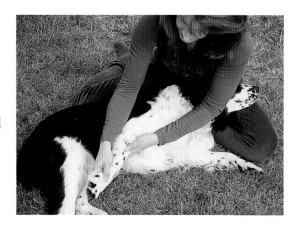

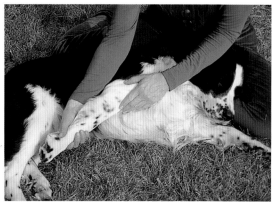

> ### THE SUPPORTING HAND
>
> The hand that holds and supports but does not move is especially important. It will create a feeling of comfort and security, and also sense any discomfort in the body part being stretched. The supporting hand should be **dynamically relaxed**.

FRONT FOOT ROTATION

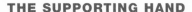

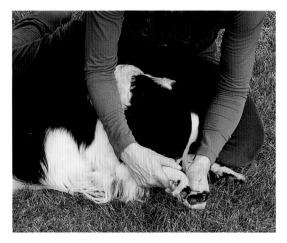

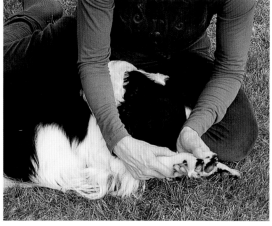

Place your supporting hand above the foot. Hold gently but firmly without gripping or squeezing. Hold the foot with the other hand.

Begin in a neutral position, then begin to rotate, tracing a circular motion. Rotate slowly and smoothly.

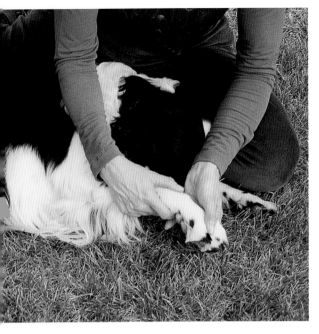

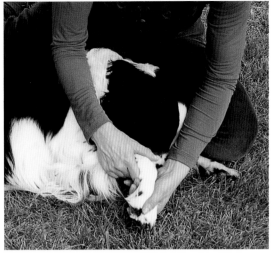

Each circular rotation should take 8-10 seconds to complete.

You may now rotate and stretch each toe.

FRONT TOE ROTATION AND STRETCHES

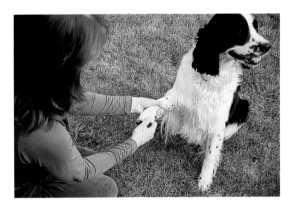

Hold the foot with one hand. Place the thumb of the other hand on top of the toe. Rotate the toe in a circular motion, taking 3-5 seconds for each rotation.

Still holding the toe, and supporting the foot, stretch the toe by leaning your body slightly rearwards, then releasing the toe back to a neutral position by sitting up again. Always be aware of the supporting and active roles of your hands.

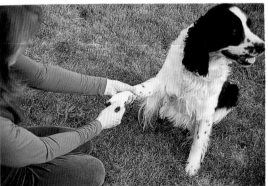

HAPPY FEET

If you know beforehand that your dog has sensitive feet, and doesn't like them to be touched, do not attempt to work on them at all for the first few sessions. Perhaps when you eventually do include them in the session, your dog will happily accept the attention.

BACK LEG

ROTATION

Hold the leg in both hands for rotation. The movement of your dog's hip joint is accomplished by moving your body with a circular motion. First, lean backwards. Next, lean sideways, bringing the leg towards the front leg. Next, lean forwards, in preparation for leaning to the other side, creating the rearward portion of the rotation. Repeat 2-3 times. This prepares him for the next step which is a slight stretch.

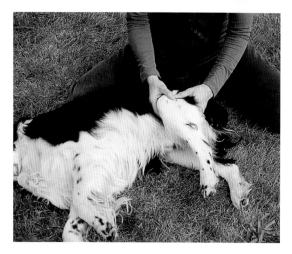

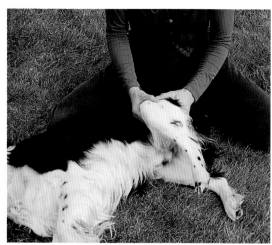

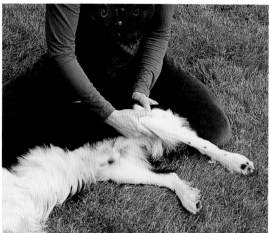

STRETCHING

Bring the leg slowly rearwards, and continue to lean your body to the side.

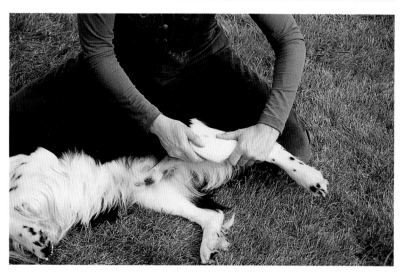

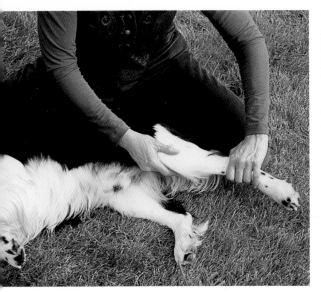

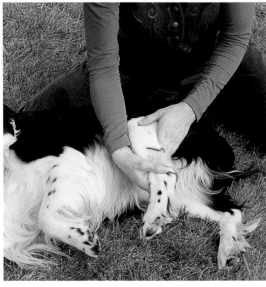

Continue to stretch as you straighten the leg, always maintaining a natural position. This picture shows maximum stretch. Hold steadily for 3-5 seconds. If your dog begins to resist, bring the leg back into a neutral position without removing your hands.

In a continuous motion make the transition from the rearward stretch to a forward stretch. Change your hand position as shown to maintain a feeling of support and continuity.

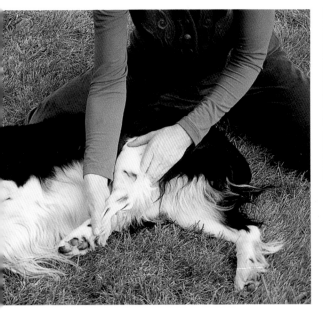

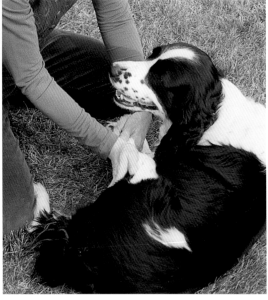

Bring the leg forwards, by leaning your body, unfolding the leg and holding the stretch. Don't try to straighten the leg, just support it in a natural position.

You may also perform these movements while sitting in front of your dog. Follow the same technique of moving your body to stretch the dog's leg.

BACK FOOT ROTATION

Place your supporting hand just above the foot and hold the foot with the other hand. Begin a range-of-motion rotation by moving your body and letting your hands become an extension of this motion. 'Listen' through your hands for signs of resistance as you rotate. End the rotation by holding the foot in a flexed position for a few seconds.

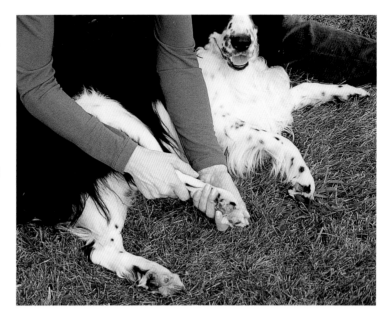

PROBLEM PREVENTION

Side-to-side and backward movement will be minimal. Don't force or try to exaggerate this. These rotations are all geared to prevent stiffness before it occurs. Prevention of problems is our main focus.

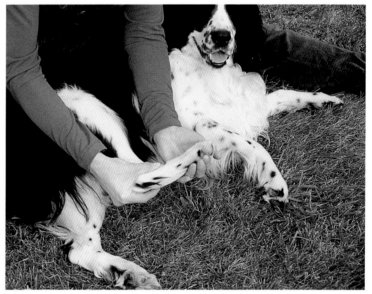

DO NOT DISTURB

It is likely that your dog has fallen asleep by now, or is in an extremely deep state of relaxation. If you need to move your body to another location for a different technique, move slowly and quietly, being careful to retain continuity. Do not bump him accidentally. Continuity is important to the dog's level of comfort, relaxation and trust, so let each technique flow from the previous one. Keep at least one hand on the dog at all times and move slowly and deliberately.

BACK TOES

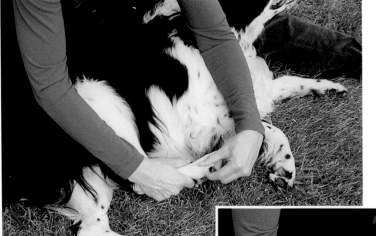

Just as you stretched the toes of the front feet, stretch the toes of the back feet. With your thumb in the top of each toe, slowly rotate, then stretch the toe by leaning slightly to the side. Release slowly.

Make a smooth transition from one toe to the next.

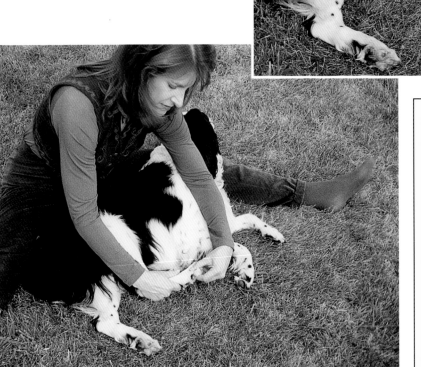

TICKLISH FEET

If your dog is reluctant to cooperate with the foot and toe techniques, just hold the foot for a moment in your hands, warming it and talking to him. His feet, like yours may be sensitive, and even ticklish. Never force a technique. It can wait until the next time. The process is important here, not the number of techniques you finish.

FRONT AND BACK LEG FULL STRETCH

To complete the side position techniques in a pleasurable finale, stretch the front leg forwards and the back leg rearwards. This is achieved by leaning forward and letting your arms change position from slightly bent to an almost straight position. Take a few seconds to go into the stretch, hold 3-5 seconds then release slowly.

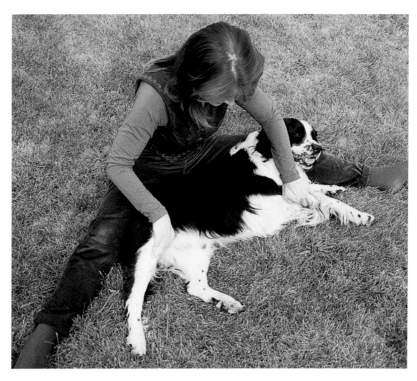

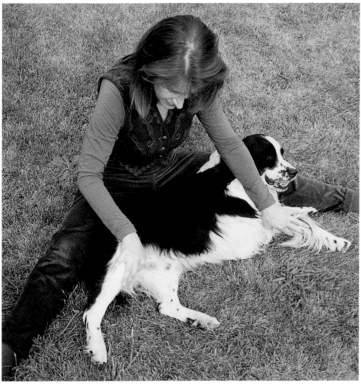

STRETCHING PLEASURE

Watch his face and listen to his breathing as you stretch. You may be rewarded with yawns, groans, and kisses if your hand happens to be within licking distance.

Many dogs instinctively know it is time to do the otherside: they will get up, stretch, and turn. You may then repeat the leg sequence on the other side.

THE NECK

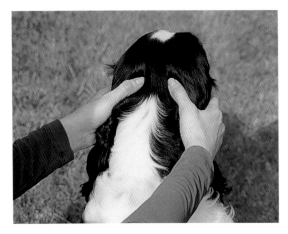

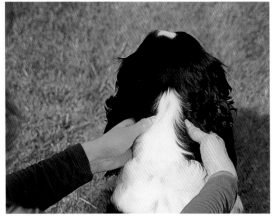

Place the thumbs at the top of your dog's neck, directly under the skull (the occipital ridge). You will feel an indentation here. The thumbs will be separated by the neck vertebra, which you may feel in the neck and the back on a thin dog, press gently and gradually inward. These points are sensitive on dogs as well as humans and may induce a feeling of pleasant relaxation. Hold for 3-5 seconds, release slowly, then place your thumbs on the next location which will be half an inch to one inch down the neck, depending on the size of the dog. Stop just above the shoulders. You may repeat this neck sequence two or three times.

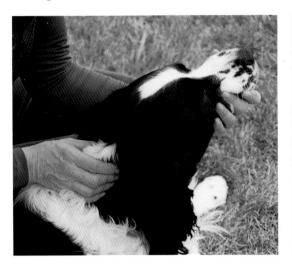

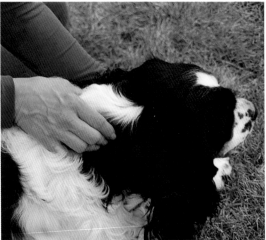

Apply the thumb and four fingers outside the big muscles on each side of your dog's neck. Hold softly but firmly. Place your other hand under his chin, and encourage him to rest his head in your hand. Bring his head upwards, towards the side, downwards, and up again towards the other side, tracing a circular motion. The neck should move smoothly without restriction, and without any hesitation on the part of the dog. Rotate once or twice in each direction. The movement is very slow.

THE EYES

UPPER EYE

With his chin resting in your cupped hand, lightly touch his head with the heel of your other hand so as not to startle him when you apply your fingertips above his eye. Feel the bony eye socket, then, beginning near the inner corner, touch lightly with the tips of your middle and ring finger, and work towards the outer corner of the eye, pressing and releasing a few points.

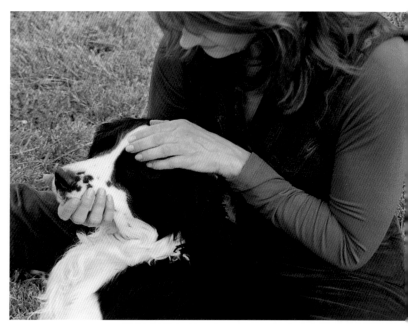

LOWER EYE

Place your thumb on the bony area under his eye, and work in the same manner towards the outer corner (this under-eye pressure is applied slightly downwards).

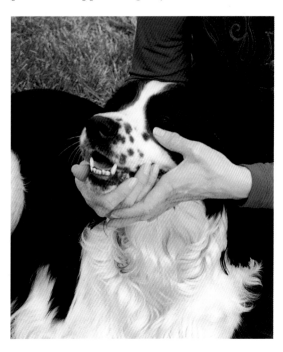

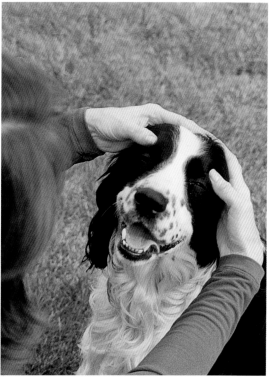

Adapt your body position and technique to work both eyes simultaneously.

THE FACE

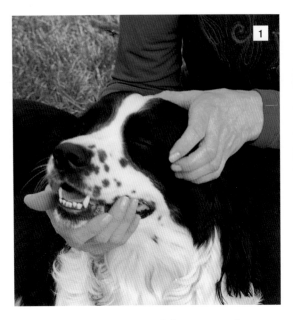

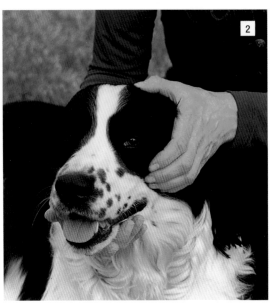

From the outer corner of the eye apply your fingertips, moving gradually down the cheek, moulding your fingers to fit the contours of the face. Work towards the jaw, and also towards the ear. These are not areas in which dogs get touched too often, so take your time and keep your hands soft and completely without tension.

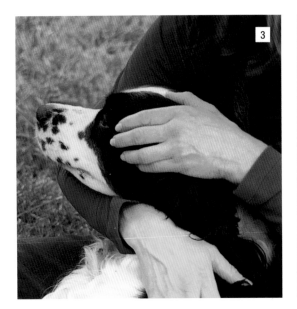

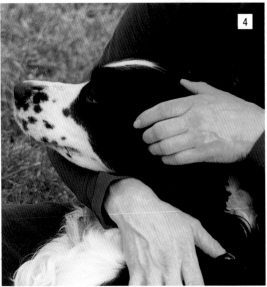

When practising these techniques you may wish to use different positions for supporting your dog; photos 1 and 2 show the dog's chin supported in a cupped hand and photos 3 and 4 show how the head can be supported in the crook of your arm.

THE MOUTH

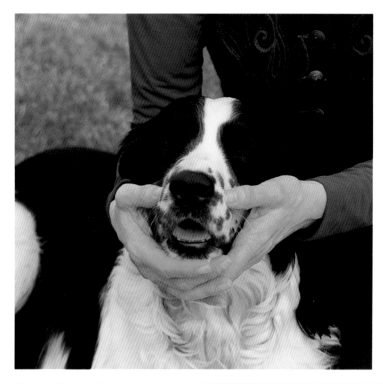

Cradle your dog's head in your hands. With your thumbs, press into the gums. You may use a slightly circular motion at each location. Work up towards the nose and back towards the eyes.

Carefully reach underneath the lips and stretch the jowls outwards slightly.

AIDING TREATMENT

Handling the mouth will make it easier to check the teeth as well as administer medication.

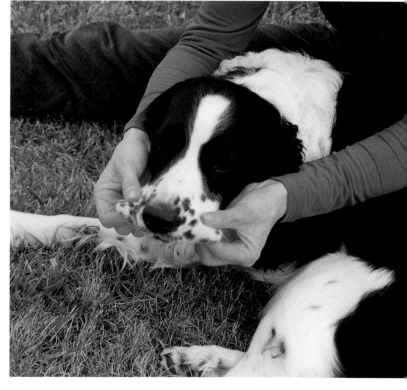

THE EARS

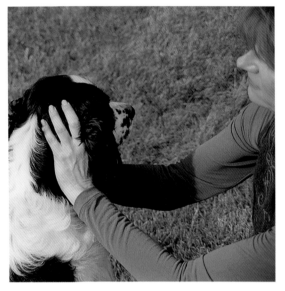

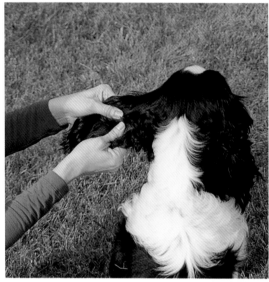

Slide your hand into position with your index finger in front of the dog's ear, your other three fingers behind the ear, and your palm against the head. Your other hand is supporting the other side of the head. Rotate the ear in each direction two or three times. You will actually be moving the skin slightly.

Now hold the ear in both hands and press from base to end, gradually pulling the ear outwards, but not enough to affect the position of the head.

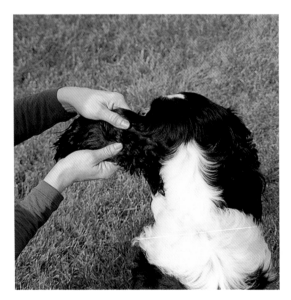

Repeat the above technique, this time drawing the ear slightly forwards.

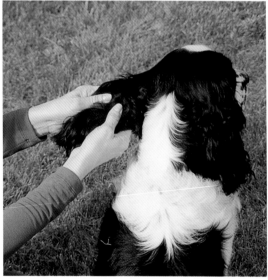

Repeat the technique again, drawing the ear rearwards.

THE TOP OF THE HEAD

Support the dog's head in your hands and apply your thumbs above his eyes, using the width of the inner corners of the eyes as a guideline for the spacing of your thumbs. Press inwards toward the skull, being careful not to slide towards the eyes. Lift your thumbs slightly but not completely, and move to the next location, which will be directly behind the first. Finish just below the occipital ridge (see first photo on p15).

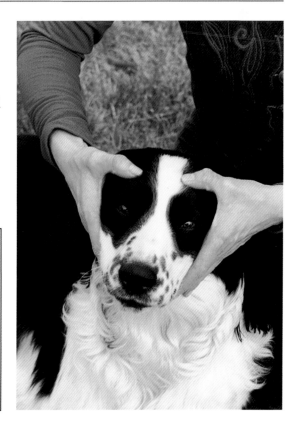

ADD VARIETY TO THE SESSIONS

You may begin or end the session with the face and head techniques. If you begin with these, continue the session by working on the neck and the back. Varying the sequence will keep you both interested, and prevent you from becoming too mechanical in your approach. You may also vary the speed and number of repetitions.

THE TAIL

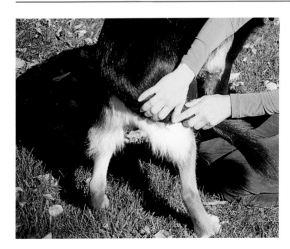

Hold the dog's tail in both hands and bring it across his body towards you. Hold for 2-3 seconds.

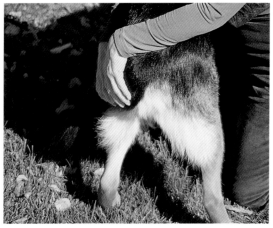

Take the tail across to the other side by adjusting your body position and the positioning of your hands.

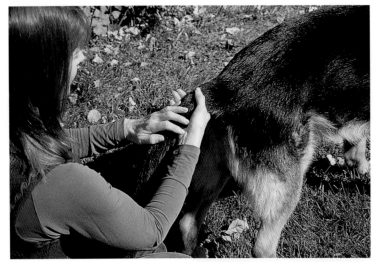

Place one hand under the tail, near the top. With the other hand on the top of the tail gently apply pressure downwards this will move the tail bones a little; the hand under the tail will simultaneously press slightly upwards.

Work your way toward the end of the tail, holding each position for 2-3 seconds.

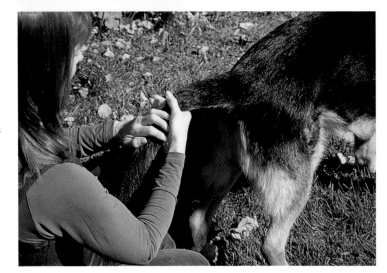

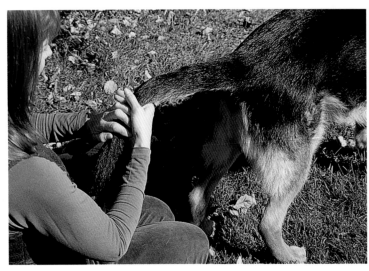

The tail treatment continues on page 22 ▶

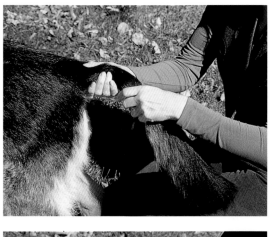
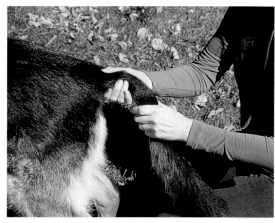
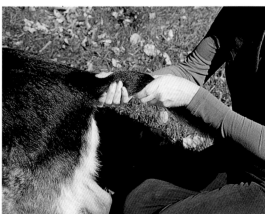
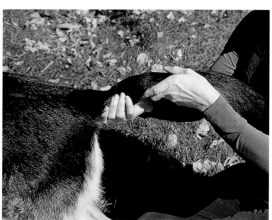

Support the underneath of the tail near the top. Hold directly below your supporting hand with your moving hand. Gradually rotate the tail sidewards, downwards, to the other side, and upwards. Rotate two to three times in each direction. Each revolution should take at least 5-7 seconds. Repeat this technique working your way towards the end of the tail.

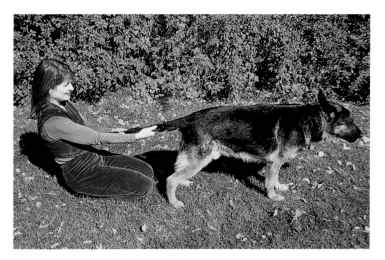

Sit directly behind the dog. Separate your hands on the tail, not holding too close to the end. The dog should be standing evenly on all four feet with the head facing the front. Begin to lean your body back slowly. Sense the dog's body. He will lean forwards to create his own stretch. Hold several seconds and release by sitting up slowly.

OLDER DOGS AND PUPPIES

Shiatsu will help older dogs stay more comfortable as their bodies age and will help injuries to heal. It is especially important to restrict vigorous activity for up to half an hour following a full body session to prevent further injury.

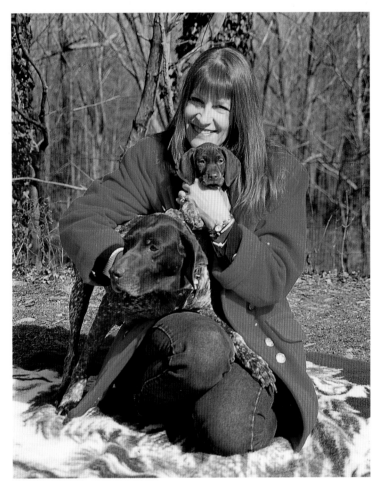

As puppies are rather unceremoniously weaned from their mothers who spend most of their day in physical contact with their offspring, shiatsu will help these babies make the adjustment to bonding with their humans.

With their soft bones and muscles, they have little need for deep pressure and long stretches. Gentle movement of their bodies will help you understand them as they grow, develop, and become more muscular.

Spend time working their feet and faces. It will be easier to groom them, and administer medication if they are accustomed to your thorough contact from puppyhood.

Since puppies have such a short attention span, a few minutes here and there rather than attempting an entire session at one sitting will be easier to accomplish. Choose a time not too close to meal time – either before or after. A good time for shiatsu would be when a puppy is a little tired and relaxed after play.

ACKNOWLEDGEMENTS

My thanks to Nancie, Ed and Alisa Giblock for my model, Max (English Springer Spaniel), to Issy Kelly and Peter Migliorato for my model, Quad (German Shepherd) and to Elaine Hollowell for my German Shorthair models.

DEDICATION

To Candy, Yukon, Sancho and Rich Dog

British Library Cataloguing-in-Publication Data.
A catalogue record for this book is available from the British Library

ISBN 0.85131.710.3

Published in Great Britain in 1998 by
J. A. Allen & Company Limited,
1 Lower Grosvenor Place, Buckingham Palace Road,
London, SW1W OEL

Design and Typesetting by Paul Saunders
Photography by Richard Aschoff
Series editor Jane Lake
Colour Separation by Tenon & Polert (H.K.) Ltd
Printed in Hong Kong by Dah Hua Printing Press Co. Ltd.